Exercises for Feeling Mindfully: Volume Seven

Mindfulness Practices for Persons with Parkinson's Disease

9/3/2014
Parkinsons Recovery
Robert Rodgers PhD

Exercises for Feeling Mindfully
Mindfulness Practices for Persons with Parkinson's Disease
Volume Seven

Contents

The Parkinsons Recovery Mindfulness Series

Realistically speaking, how can the intense level of stress that aggravates the symptoms of Parkinson's disease be calmed? Better yet, how can they be quieted? My research over the past decade reveals that using your mind to drop the stress level down a notch or two always backfires. When you tell yourself:

- *Settle down!*
- *Take it easy!*
- *Stop being so stressed out!*

The stress level ratchets up, not down. Attempts to force the stress and anxiety levels to adjust downward induce an internally generated stress. They pile more stress on top of an excess of stress that already exists. There are certainly a sufficient number of external generators of stress in every one's life. Why infuse more stress that you create yourself, even with the best of intentions?

If the mind is not a useful technique to reduce stress, what is? The most eloquent answer I have for you is to become more mindful of what is experienced in the present moment. Becoming more mindful shifts you into the experience of the "now" which in itself is less stressful (unless you have been kidnapped by terrorists!).

It is stressful to anticipate events you imagine will occur in the future. The events we imagine rarely happen. Does this ring true for you? We all create unnecessary stress in our lives by how and where we focus our thoughts and attention.

It is stressful to agonize over the past. When we think about the past, we are much more likely to think about unpleasant experiences that induce stress. The past event itself was traumatic enough. Yet, we insist on reliving the trauma over and over again through our memories. It seems some of us just can't get enough stress in our lives.

The problem with upping the ante on stress levels is that – as you well know – symptoms of Parkinson's disease become worse. When you are not as stressed, your symptoms are far less problematic.

I have reached one solid conclusion from my ten years of research on Parkinson's disease. Symptoms will drive you crazy when you are stressed and are far less problematic when stress is under control.

Now, if you can't use your mind to become more mindful (which creates added stress in itself) how in the world can you quiet down a frantic lifestyle? I have concluded that the simplest and most effective solution to reducing stress levels is to become more mindful.

The transformation is possible step by step through these simple exercises you can do anywhere, anytime of the day. The Parkinsons Recovery mindfulness exercises are designed to focus your attention on the present moment as attention on either the past or the future is diverted. A renewed focus on the present moment reduces stress levels. Mindfulness is a lifestyle that will reduce stresses in your life if you set the intention to take a mindfulness practice seriously.

I recommend that you practice each of the exercises for a week or longer. Incorporate each practice into your regular routines and habits. Attempts to do all of the exercises simultaneously will likely induce more stress which – obviously – is contrary to the intent of a successful mindfulness program.

Give each exercise a little time and space. Invite the stresses in your life to dissipate. Allow the experience of each practice to engulf you. In so doing, watch the stresses in your life dip down to new lows along with a concurrent relief of any and all symptoms that you have currently been experiencing.

This volume is one out of nine I have developed to support the recovery of persons who currently experience neurological symptoms. A full listing of the Parkinsons Recovery Mindfulness themes follows:

Exercises for Feeling Mindfully
Mindfulness Practices for Persons with Parkinson's Disease
Volume Seven

Volume 1: Exercises for Seeing Mindfully

Volume 2: Exercises for Hearing Mindfully

Volume 3: Exercises for Noticing Mindfully

Volume 4: Exercises for Doing Mindfully

Volume 5: Exercises for Eating Mindfully

Volume 6: Exercises for Thinking Mindfully

Volume 7: Exercises for Feeling Mindfully

Volume 8: Exercises for Being Mindfully

Volume 9: Exercises for Intending Mindfully

Robert Rodgers, PhD

Parkinsons Recovery

www.parkinsonsrecovery.me

Olympia, Washington

Notice Suffering

My mindfulness challenge for you this week is to become fully and completely attentive to the suffering of other persons. Let me make something absolutely clear at the outset. The invitation is not that you suffer yourself. Rather, become aware and sensitive to the suffering of other persons.

Suffering can come in rather extreme packages. We are certainly all aware of the suffering of individuals who are seriously ill and in pain. Suffering can also assume milder forms. There can be many nuances of suffering in the tone of a person's voice, in their expressions or even in the way they may hesitate or stumble over the words they speak. During each and every encounter with another individual, become fully attentive and aware of all suffering that may be evident.

Some examples may help flesh out the idea behind the challenge this week.

- *You are driving in your car down the street. A person driving in their car behind you decides that they need to drive a couple of inches behind your back bumper. Look in the mirror. Examine the expression on their face. Sink in to what may be going on with the person who is hot on your tail. There is obviously suffering present.*

6

- *You are standing in a line waiting to pay for groceries. The person behind you is obviously agitated. Their body is tense and contorted. They are eager to pass through the line very, very quickly. Look. Notice the expression on their face. Be attentive to what is going on with them in the present moment.*

- *You are sitting at the dinner table when a family member blurbs out an emotional outburst. Pay close attention to their ever changing feelings as they unfold over the course of the outburst. Suffering can settle in for a spell and - all of a sudden – vanish in a flash. Observe any indications of irritation, flashes of anger and little flares of frustration that slip out uncontrollably. Take delight in a release from the suffering which may be accompanied by a funny joke. The shifts can be shocking and nuances flabbergasting.*

- *You are listening to your favorite radio show when a listener calls in to rant. Extend your assessment of suffering to people on the radio who rant. You can hear the suffering expressed in their voices.*

Suffering is ever-present in every one's life. We do not have to be licensed detectives to confront it firsthand in ourselves or in others.

Be aware of what suffering looks like. How does it feel inside your body when you connect from a deep place inside of you with the suffering of another? Is there a unique sensation in your physical body that emerges? Does the suffering you encounter assume an intensity that ranges from mild to severe? Or, is the intensity even handed and reserved?

Make no judgments. Simply observe. Be mindful of each and every encounter you have with a person who is suffering in the moment.

When you observe suffering - and you are likely to observe it often over the course of just one day - do a quick assessment of its character, intensity and extensiveness.

Most of us (myself included!) prefer to run away from suffering. Turn that fear around this week. Become more and more sensitive and attentive to the suffering of each person you encounter. Please keep in mind - as I said at the outset – please do not take on the suffering of others. It is not yours to have. Simply become observant of the suffering of others and leave it at that. This exercise should not stress you out!

Deeper Implications of Suffering

You may well have been thinking to yourself these past few days -

> *"The mindfulness challenge this week to be attentive to suffering has not been any fun at all. What a horrible idea!"*

Some of you might have decided to set this particular mindfulness assignment aside and either revisit a previous challenge or take a much deserved vacation from mindfulness challenges. Why in the world did I suggest that you become attentive to suffering?

Suffering, as it turns out, is an extra burden we create all on our own that applies an overlay of mental angst and emotional distress on top of physical pain. Suffering is not required or necessary. It is something that we impose on ourselves that amplifies the physical pain.

How many times have you seen an individual, particularly those that you love, suffer. You think to yourself or even say to them -

> *"Stop! Get over it. Get on with your life."*

How many times have you had that thought or expressed it to another person?

Permit me to introduce a rambling tirade that imposes additional challenges that are quite necessary. Dealing with the physical pain taken alone is a formidable challenge in itself. Imposing the additional burdens of suffering is overwhelming and unmanageable. Perhaps the following tirade may sound vaguely familiar to you?

> "This is the second painful cramp that I've had in my right calf this week. Yuck! This time I'm sure it's going to get worse just like it did before when this happened several weeks ago. This cramp is more than I can stand. What in the world is wrong with me? First there was the problem of tremor, then unsteadiness and now cramping? What's really going on? Oh my God. Perhaps the cramping that I'm experiencing right now is something really, really serious. Maybe the reason I'm cramping is that I have a brain tumor. Maybe I have cancer. Maybe it's something really serious like a stroke is about to unfold. Oh my God."

The tirade above gives you a flavor of the irrational impositions that we too often attach to physical pain. This cacophony of worries and frets adds a thick layer of anxiety which is entirely unnecessary and unwarranted.

Adding the overlay of suffering makes the pain so much acute and troubling.

All of the statements and thoughts in this tirade are fabrications of my imagination. They impose additional burdens that need not be assumed. Why? They never existed in the first place. The person in the rant did not have a stroke! They do not have cancer!

It is recommended to set suffering aside when the rattle trap of negative thoughts creep into your head.

> *"Oh, I'm sure my reasoning is obviously ridiculous. Let me just place this tirade on the top shelf of my 'stupid and silly thoughts' kitchen cabinet. I can always take out these worries tomorrow if I choose and enjoy suffering over again if I choose. I do not have to give up the thrill of my ranting!"*

Place the tirade of suffering inside the imaginary cabinet shelf. Shut the cabinet door. Of course you may want to re-visit the thoughts tomorrow, especially if you are eager to find a little pleasure out of revisiting the rant. Admittedly, we can all derive pleasure from suffering. Most people, however, discover that once the ranting thoughts have been locked up in the cabinet, they have no need to re-visit them.

Once the overlay of suffering has been locked up, forgotten and dissolved, initiate a dialogue with the cramping in your right calf or your right thigh or your left thigh or with whatever difficulties you might currently be experiencing.

- *What's up here?*
- *What's going on?*
- *How does that discomfort actually feel?*
- *Does it come and go?*
- *Does it have intensity that fluctuates?*
- *Is it sharp in character?*
- *Is it dull?*
- *What does that discomfort actually feel like in the moment?*

When people wipe away the overlay of suffering that they imposed on the pain and the discomfort, guess what? The pain and discomfort lesson. You begin to feel a little better. The pain is not as acute or as bothersome.

I know you probably think I have got it all backwards. It would seem more logical to predict that when you pay closer attention to pain it should get worse. Right? Not true.

If you really sink into what is going on with your body, you can not only get an accurate fix of the character of the discomfort but get some help with determining its root

12

cause. Once you get a few good clues about the cause, you are finally in a position to do something about it.

To summarize - suffering is unnecessary. It is something that we impose on ourselves that creates misery and accentuates pain. Symptoms become significantly worse when we add the unnecessary ingredient of suffering.

It is easiest to notice the suffering in others which is the reason for the challenge this week. If your experience has been like mine, it is overwhelming to realize how much suffering people create for themselves. Shift that awareness to yourself. Why not take suffering out of the equation? It is not helping!

To summarize, when you impose suffering on top of the pain, gather together all rambling thoughts of suffering. Place the entire tirade inside your imaginary kitchen cabinet of "stupid and silly thoughts" shut the door.

Once suffering is out of the picture you have the opportunity to be more mindful and attentive to the signals your body is sending moment to moment. Disengage suffering from the physical character of symptoms. Your body is always trying to send messages to you moment to moment. Put suffering aside. This does not eliminate the pain, but it makes it much more tolerable.

Mindful Waiting

The mindfulness challenge this week will be triggered each and every time you find yourself waiting in a line for service. A companion challenge I extend (if and only if you choose to accept it) is to stand in the longest line when you have a choice. Whatever line you choose, be attentive to what is happening inside your body as you patiently wait.

- *Relax all of the tension that you may be holding deep within your tissues and muscles.*
- *Pay attention to how you stand as you wait - on one foot or both feet?*
- *Notice how you are breathing.*
- *Quiet your thoughts of irritation toward the person ahead of you who is taking longer than necessary.*

If impatience emerges, if your mind becomes noisy with angry thoughts - silence them. Re-direct your attention and focus to your physical body. Become aware of the heat that rises from your skin or the cold that sinks into your bones. What signals does your body send as you wait?

Most importantly, relax all of the tension in your muscles whether that tension be in your

- *Calf muscles*
- *Thigh muscles*
- *Chest muscles*
- *Neck muscles*
- *Eyebrows*
- *Ears*

Become aware of all the tension in your body from head to toe as you patiently and mindfully wait for the service that you seek.

Notice your body settling down into a state of calm. Become aware of how it is possible to reverse neurological symptoms as you calm down the irritation that sizzles inside the tissues of your body.

1. Wait patiently
2. Wait mindfully
3. Shift your focus from irritation and impatience to a patient practice of mindfulness.

May you relish the challenge of waiting patiently in long lines this week.

15

Deeper Meaning Behind Mindful Waiting

There is no question about it. We all carve out ruts of irritation in our neurological pathways. I use the word ruts intentionally. We all become irritated over and over, oftentimes at the very same circumstances that, for whatever reason, drive us up the wall and make us crazy.

The same patterns of behavior are repeated frequently. Such patterned and habitual responses create an elaborate infrastructure of blockages that obstruct the function of our neurological system. We carve out ruts in our sensitive neurological pathways much like the ruts and holes in the dirt roads created by the pioneers who traveled across the Oregon trail in the eighteen hundreds.

It does not take much to re-enter these well-established ruts in any neurological system. They aggravate the neurological challenges of Parkinson's disease.

The mindfulness challenge this week is to pave new neurological roadways that remove the irritants to our sensitive neurological system. When we engage in negative thoughts like,

> *"Why can't that idiot in front of me in line hurry up and get done? I've got something important to do and I'm going to be late."*

The body's neurological system does in fact become irritated as we process the signals of irritation and anger triggered by the same neurological pathways full of ruts.

How do you create new neural pathways that calm the neurological system rather than upset it? Learn how to offer a different response to situations that are likely to irritate you such as standing in long lines. Instead of accessing the same neurological ruts (as you become impatient) access new pathways. Calm your body by focusing on the full context of your present circumstances. Use your intention to offer a different response to these circumstances.

Shift your awareness from one of outward projection to inward reflection. As you wait in line, breathe and notice the deliciousness of what it really feels like to take on the critical source of life itself – oxygen. .

- *Relax all the tension in your body as you wait.*
- *Notice how you stand.*
- *Observe where you stand.*
- *Re-position your weight if it helps you become more comfortable.*
- *Silence all angry thoughts of people ahead of you who may simply be having a bad day.*

As you engage a new response to a circumstance that can be irritating you receive the added benefit of forging new

17

neurological pathways. As your stress level dissolves, notice how symptoms you might have been experiencing are not as troublesome. Better yet, perhaps they will not even get activated. A body that is calm and stress free is not capable (or interested) in creating neurological difficulties for you.

Switch on a mindfulness practice as you wait –

- *Become aware of each and every sensation*
- *Look up at the ceiling.*
- *Look down at the floor.*
- *Notice the walls.*
- *Notice the texture of the walls.*
- *Appreciate the colors on the walls.*
- *Smile at the people who wait with you.*
- *Hear the sounds.*
- *Smell the scents.*

Take in sensually everything in your surroundings. Notice how delicious it can be to become aware of your surroundings.

Mindfulness practices do result in an alleviation of neurological symptoms. The more you practice mindfulness, the more you will be delighted with the result. We are the ones that manifest our own destiny. Make it so this week.

Just Say Yes

Over three decades ago, First Lady Nancy Reagan launched and supported a program to help children stop using drugs. The program was known as "Just Say No." My mindfulness invitation for you this week is just the reverse of Nancy Reagan's program. My invitation is to

> *"Just Say Yes"*

To everything that happens and anything that is suggested to you.

I realize this exercise sounds quite outrageous. There are obviously some suggestions that will obviously not be in your best interest or even in the best interest of the person making the suggestion. If the suggestion might result in a risk to life or safety, suggest an alternative or diversion. If, for example you are working with a child or a grandchild and they want to do something that obviously might create some risk to their safety, divert their attention rather than immediately saying:

> *"No, you will get hurt if you do just that."*

It may be very difficult in some situations to simply say yes. In such situations, I invite you to consider the possibility of smiling. Simply be present and pleasant. When a person suggests an idea that you find to be particularly aversive or distasteful for whatever reason, simply smile. Be pleasant. Do not engage or initiate any disagreement. Do not argue.

When you say "yes" you have an opportunity to get in touch with what is going on with your energy and your feelings. You will discover the experience is very different from situations when you wind up saying "no".

- *That is not a good idea.*
- *That is not a good plan.*

Instead of saying "no", offer a simple, unqualified response. It does not matter what the person says or thinks or has argued. Just say yes. Saying "no" is habitual for many people. When some people do not agree they offer no response whatsoever. Instead, make saying "Yes" your habitual and immediate response to everyone you encounter. Experience what happens to your energy. You can always say "No" later if necessary.

Deeper Meaning Behind Saying "Yes"

What is the deeper meaning behind an exercise that challenges you with always saying "Yes" no matter what is suggested? It is the case that persons in some occupations tend to be oppositional. Certainly that is the job of lawyers who have been trained to argue and dispute any claim. Certainly that is the job of academics whose training is to find fatal flaws in studies.

Why did I personally decide to become qualified to be become an academic and receive academic appointments at large, state universities? The real reason I think, in retrospect, was job security. I did not want to be poor. I did not want to be dependent on others. I wanted to be able to take care of myself. I thought this was going to be my job for life.

What really happened? I resigned my position as a full, tenured professor at the University of Kentucky a decade ago. The reason of job security was not a good enough reason to continue doing the work of a professor.

Perhaps there might have been other reasons for pursuing the work of a professor? I could have wanted to earn a PhD because I loved teaching or research. In retrospect, however, those were not the true reasons. I did not want anyone to be in a position to fire me arbitrarily.

What I learned about the work is that it is dominated with arguments and judgments. When studies are reviewed every aspect of the research is criticized (and many of the criticisms are unjustified). People who review studies for publication rarely say "Yes".

Doing work that is oppositional and argumentative takes us up into our heads. By way of custom and habit we rattle about one possibility after another before we either say "yes" or "no". We are always pondering. We are always evaluating. We are always looking for flaws. That argumentative approach – that set of skills – has a very different feel to it, a very different energy than the energy associated with simply saying yes. It gave me little joy to life a life where I was always saying "no" and hearing "no" so I quit my university job that was guaranteed for a lifetime.

What has happened when you said "yes" to situations these past few days, situations where you normally would have paused and said "no"? Is it possible that saying yes has alerted you to instantly realize your real answer is a clear and unequivocal "no". In other words, by saying "yes" you immediately realized,

"Oh, heavens, this is definitely something I would never really want to do."

22

Alternatively, you might have spent hour after hour pontificating whether it would be a good decision or not. By simply saying "yes", your body has told you there is no way you should pursue that possibility. You knew at the outset it was a lousy idea. By saying "yes", you prevented yourself from wasting all the time evaluating what to do.

Do you dismiss opportunities out of hand because of prior commitments? Perhaps the reason why you say "No" to doing something that you would love to do is because you have already made a prior commitment.

- Do you immediately say no because of those commitments?
- Do you place a high value on loyalty and commitment?
- Do prior commitments always take priority over any new, exciting opportunity?
- Do you always dismiss opportunities out of hand because of prior commitments?

  "No. Sorry. I can't go on that 3 day, all expenses paid trip to Hawaii because I promised to make a chocolate cake for my Uncle."

Really?

Perhaps saying "yes" will alert you to the endless hours that you spend in your head agonizing over decisions (just like a hamster who spins around and around and around its hamster wheel pondering, figuring, assessing and mind tripping). The obvious answer to some opportunities is to respond with an immediate yes.

"Of course that is something I would love to do."

Just saying "yes" offers an opportunity to examine the energy behind resistance in contrast to the energy behind moving forward in life.

What does this all have to do with experiencing the symptoms of Parkinson's disease? Many people are focused on the symptoms. They say "No" to the symptoms continuously throughout the day.

- *No to the fact that this left arm happens to be tremoring day after day.*
- *No to the fact that I can't swallow as I used to swallow one year ago.*
- *No to the fact that I can't talk loudly and clearly.*
- *No to the fact that I have pain in my right thigh.*
- *No, no, no, no.*

The focus is on the negative "no" rather than that positive "Yes" to living life to its fullest.

The amazing discovery that I have made over the past decade of my research on Parkinson's disease is that when individuals pursue an activity that they truly love,

24

symptoms seem to dissolve. It actually does not seem to matter what the activity is.

- *I've seen people in wheelchairs who, when afforded the opportunity to line dance, slowly got out of their wheel chair, held on to another person and by George, line danced up and down the dance floor.*

- *I've seen people who had serious symptoms associated with the diagnosis of Parkinson's disease who were able to play championship ping pong games without showing any evidence of symptoms whatsoever.*

- *I've seen painters with troublesome symptoms who – once they launch a painting project – do not experience any tremoring or any other symptoms whatsoever.*

In activity after activity I hear report after report from persons who say,

> *"I don't seem to have any symptoms whatsoever when I play with my granddaughter or grandson or son or daughter."*

I invite you to seriously ponder what you genuinely love to do. What haven't you been doing recently that you always loved to do in the past? Why not focus on the 'yes' of your life? Start doing what it is that you truly love to do.

When you begin to spend and allocate your thinking energy on the "Yes" to living life to the fullest, problematic symptoms will become less and less worrisome and bothersome. Saying "yes" has a far more energetic charge than saying "no".

Saying "no" creates a diffusion of energy. It creates equivocality. It creates hesitation. It paralyzes. We do not move forward when we always stop to evaluate and question. We do not move forward in our life's purpose when we say "no". In contrast, we always get a surge of delicious energy when we say "yes".

Clearly you don't want to say "yes" to everything. That is not the point of this mindfulness exercise. The point of this particular mindfulness challenge is to tease out the difference between when you do say "Yes" and when you do say "No." When you shift your "no" responses to "yes" responses you receive an infusion of high energy. You get to enjoy pursing your passions. There is nothing stopping you when you are in the habit of saying "yes." You get more energy. You have more fun when you say "yes" to life. You lose energy and get depressed when you say "no."

Of course symptoms may still be present here and there, but the focus is no longer on symptoms. The focus is on the life that you choose to lead. May you have a magnificent time with the challenge of the week as you continue to say "Yes to Life" now and forever more.

Smile

My mindfulness challenge for you this week is to smile each and every time you see a reflection of yourself in a mirror or perhaps even in a windowpane. Invite yourself to smile even if the image that you see of yourself shows a person who is sad or neutral in their expression.

You may say to yourself,

> *"What just a minute Rodgers, you're telling me that if I'm feeling really low and down in the dumps I'm supposed to pretend as though I'm happy, I have to put a happy face on? That's not genuine. I'm a person who thinks it's important to be truthful about who I am and how I am feeling."*

I say to you this perspective is all well and good. I honor you for the authenticity that you treasure near and dear to your heart. However, research shows that smiles transform moods.

There is a technology known as Laughter Yoga. Ever heard of it? The practice consists of people sitting around a circle who laugh. Jokes are not even a part of this therapy. People literally just force themselves to laugh. When they start the exercise I can assure you everyone is not feeling in a positive mood. When they finish, everyone is surprised about how good they feel. Forcing smiles through forced laughter does transform moods.

When I walk down the sidewalks in downtown Olympia, I pass many people. I can assure you that when I pass by an individual who has a smile on their face, I feel yummy inside. It really transforms whatever mood state I might currently be in. I also know that when I walk in downtown Olympia, Washington with a smile on my face, each person that I pass by also has a transformation. They usually begin smiling as well. I affect others and at the same time have a positive impact on my own mood in the moment.

In summary, each time you see an image of yourself, whether in a mirror or a reflection in a window or any reflection from any source – even if it is in water – look at yourself and smile. You will be amazed at what difference it can make with how you are feeling in the moment. Become mindful of your smiling acuity. It will make a difference on how you get through each and every day.

Deeper Implications Behind Smiling

How has your practice of mindful smiling been coming along this week? Have you noticed some resistance to the challenge? Have you resisted the challenge of smiling when you were feeling down in the dumps? I have some additional incentives that I want to offer, especially to those of you who may find the challenge to smile as frequently as possible throughout the day to be problematic.

Research shows that smiling has a number of unbelievable benefits.

- *Smiling lowers blood pressure.*
- *Smiling enhances the immune system.*
- *Smiling releases endorphins, the natural painkillers.*
- *Smiling is a natural anti-depressant.*
- *Smiling facilitates the production of serotonin.*

Best of all, people who make it a habit to smile live seven years longer than people who prefer frowns over smiles.

It also turns out that people perceive individuals who smile to be younger and more attractive. The perception is also that people who smile are more successful and someone others would like to get to know better. All in all this is an impressive list of advantages.

Might I remind you, smiling costs nothing. No doctors are required. No visit to a healthcare professional is necessary. Smiling is something you can do anytime of the day; morning, afternoon and evening. It is a divine gift that you can give to yourself anytime.

Yes, it does make other people feel better when they see us smiling and happy. It also enhances our own mood. Best of all smiling nurtures our body into being able to produce dopamine naturally. No prescription medication or supplement is required when we have that wonderful ability to smile our way throughout life.

Compliments

The challenge I cordially extend to you this week is to offer a compliment to an individual at least one time (if not two times) each day. The individual can be a friend or family member. Better yet the individual can be a total stranger. Let me explain the purpose of this particular challenge. .

To become totally and completely mindful each and every moment means we are aware of our thoughts and feelings in the present moment; not yesterday and not tomorrow, but now. Some of the feelings in the present moment are untoward, ugly and depressing. We feel an energy that drags us down into the bottom of a very, very deep valley of darkness. We feel lousy from head to toe.

Other thoughts elicit feelings of elation and excitement. We are happy that we are alive and in a body that is able to function. Thoughts and feelings are continuously changing from gloom and doom to happy and optimistic moment to moment.

Let me give an example that applies to my own situation. I am walking in downtown Olympia. I pass one person who is obese. They are very overweight. I think to myself,

"Oh my God, that person is so horribly fat."

What does that thought do to me? It sinks me into a very dark place. My energy deflates.

> *"Why am I thinking that thought about that person who may be an angel in disguise?"*

When I examine that judgmental thought I realize I am thinking this thought because I was on the scale this morning and noticed that I had upped the ante a couple of pounds since the day before. In other words, I am judging that person not because of who they are, but because of who I am.

Some thoughts have a debilitating impact on our ability to feel good about ourselves and to feel good about being in our body. Other thoughts do just the reverse.

The challenge to become mindful about our judgments as contrasted to compliments is, first of all, to become aware of what each thought does to our inner most physiological response. Better yet, let's set the intention to make public any and all thoughts that we have about others that are truly and completely complimentary.

When I walk downtown Olympia, oftentimes I have thoughts that are really quite magnificent. I see a man and I think to myself,

> *"That man dresses immaculately. My God!"*

I see a woman who has beautiful hair and I think to myself,

> *"That is the most gorgeous red I have ever seen in my life."*

I see another woman, she is walking down the sidewalk and I think to myself,

> *"That dress looks magnificent on that individual."*

I see a man. He is dressed casually. He has a dog with him who is the most eager and welcoming dog I've seen in a long time. I think to myself,

> *"That's a magnificent companion for any man to have."*

We all have these types of thoughts all the time. What do we typically do with those thoughts? What do I do with those thoughts? I keep them inside. I smile to the person. I pass by them. They never hear the compliment.

The mindfulness challenge of the week then is, once you have the thought, once the thought is heartfelt, to stop and simply tell the person what it is that you have been thinking as you were passing by them (or when you saw them).

I have practiced this challenge myself over the past week and found that it has a magnificent impact on my own energy level. I have seen a waitress who has served me a dinner and I thought to myself,

> *"She has the most magnificent smile I have ever seen in my life."*

I pause to myself and think, if I say that to this particular individual, are they going to think it's a come-on? And I hesitate, I think,

> *"Oh, that's not my intention. I want nothing other than just to let her know about my thought. I simply want her to receive the compliment, the thought that I had about her most magnificent smile is just that - nothing more and nothing less."*

After hesitating, I make the decision. I'm going to tell her. So, I do. The response is so, so fantastic. I know, that through that simple statement, I have made that individual's day. She will go home and she will tell her family,

> *"Do you know what I was told today?"*

And do you know what happens then? Her family then says,

> *"You didn't know that?"*

You see, our simple compliments have a profound impact on other people. More importantly and for purposes of this challenge, they have profound impact on us. And that is - I want to say – the reason to actually make this a regular practice. It helps us energize our life force. It helps us feel good about ourselves. It helps us shift a low-level frequency and energy straight up to a sky-high frequency which is where health and wellness resides.

When you have the thought, simply make sure it is heartfelt. When you say it, the person will get the compliment and absorb its true significance. So, why not each and every day, at least once or twice, offer a compliment to a family member, friend or better yet a stranger?

Not all will be received. Some will be rebuffed. It is of course possible that some people will expect that you are begging for some kind of an exchange. They might suspect you are offering the compliment because you expect something in return.

Yes, this is all certainly true. But when the person takes in and fully receives a compliment, you help yourself return to balance and reverse whatever symptoms you might currently experience. Each compliment you give is a golden opportunity to feel better in the moment. Each moment adds up to a lifetime.

Try it out. You will like the outcome. I certainly have.

Deeper Meaning Behind Compliments

How are the compliments going this week for you? Have you noticed a difference between offering compliments to an individual who is a stranger as contrasted to an individual who is an intimate friend or family member? Oftentimes there is a marked difference.

Persons that we know well often do not receive compliments from us. Why? There are many reasons we withhold compliments to the people we love dearly. We say to ourselves,

> *"I've told them that a thousand times."*

Or, we do not notice the positive attributes of the person. Rather, we tend to notice more of the negative aspects of that person that tend to drive us up the wall of frustration. The compliments in most relationships slowly fizzle off. It will however shift a relationship when saying what is positive and appreciated about any loved one comes from your heart.

There is a second dimension to this challenge. Some compliments that we offer to others are based on a temporary characteristic of the person. By that I mean, we compliment their hair today which is a beautiful red color but in just a few years their hair may become gray. Or, the face may be quite gorgeous today but a few wrinkles may sneak in over a few months because of dehydration. Some of the characteristics that we admire in others today are temporary. They may no longer be present in a month, or year or decade. We are all in bodies that age over time.

There is another type of compliment that can have a profound impact. This particular compliment takes the following form:

> *"Because of what you just did (or said) I feel absolutely magnificent."*

When you say how you feel in response to something a person has just done in the moment, you have just offered a compliment that the person cannot cast aside, ignore or dismiss. When offering a compliment consider prefacing it with:

> *"I feel..."*

Then fill in the blank.

> *"I feel exhilarated when I am with you right now."*
>
> *"I feel so happy hearing you say that."*
>
> *"I feel..."*

However you feel, simply state it. Then tell the person why you feel that way.

Remember - each time you vocalize a compliment to another you are shifting your energy to the place of health and wellness. You are increasing the ability of your body to heal. Positive thoughts yield positive outcomes. Kind words to another are a profound gift. They create wealth in your own heart which is the source of all healing. And, at the same time you have offer an unsolicited healing to another person.

Touch

My invitation for you this week is to become aware and sensitive of touch.

- *What does it feel like to touch objects?*
- *What does it feel like to touch people?*
- *What does it really feel like when you are "touched" by another person?*

Each time you are touched, whether it is because somebody brushed you by accident or somebody intentionally placed their hand on your shoulder, become aware and sensitive to how it feels inside your body when you are touched. Does it feel:

- *Soft*
- *Warm*
- *Cozy*
- Loving
- *Tender*

Or does the touch feel:

- *Abrasive*
- *Aggressive*
- *Sharp*
- *Edgy*
- *Unpleasant*

Each time you are touched, step back. Pause for five or ten seconds. Ask yourself,

> *"How did it feel when I was just touched by someone else?"*

Turn that assignment around. Each time you touch either a person or an object, do the very same thing.

> *"How did it feel when I just touched someone else?"*

Do the same quick assessment when you touch objects:

1. If you pick up a fork, how does the fork feel to you?
2. If you are washing a glass in the sink, how does it feel to touch that glass?
3. If you are holding a book to read, how does the book feel when it is touched by your hands?
4. If you are placing your hand inside the hand of another that you love, how does it feel inside your body at the moment when contact is made?

For each and every physical contact that you make, pause ever so effortlessly and briefly. Acknowledge when you pause how it feels when either you are touched or you touch another object or another person.

Become mindful. Become aware each and every moment of each and every experience of physical contact.

- *Is it tender?*
- Is it sweet?
- *Is it loving?*

Or, is it so quick and abrasive that it is not noticed or even acknowledged?

Deeper Meaning Behind Touch

What is the deeper meaning behind becoming aware and sensitive to touch? When we make physical contact with another person who is disconnected and detached, when there is touching but no consciousness associated with the touch - what comes back to us from that other living being is the same: detachment, disconnection and distance.

When we touch another living being with compassion, when the touch is "mindful" - what returns to us is the same: love, compassion and a deep connection. When I say "living being" I'm not just talking about persons.

Many of you are well aware of what it means to touch an animal; a dog, a cat or a horse. Horses, cats and dogs are no different than humans; when we touch an animal tenderly and lovingly, what returns back to us is the very same delicious energy that they project.

There is a deeper meaning to the "touching" exercise. To what extent are you mindfully connected in a loving way to your own body moment to moment?

- *Are you disconnected from your own body?*
- *Are you disassociated from your own body?*
- *Do you refuse to send loving energy to every cell of your body?*
- *Are you angry at your body?*

42

- *Are you furious at what your body is doing to you?*

Each time you have those thoughts, they convey an energy to every cell of your body that is not in your best and highest good.

What happens when you touch your own body? What is the experience when you hold your own hands? Is that done tenderly or is it done out of fear and anxiety?

What happens when you touch your knee? Is that done with disconnection, without any knowledge of the fact that you are touching your knee, or as you touch your knee with your hand, do you do so with intention, love and compassion? Do you transmit loving energy to each and every cell in your knee?

How we touch objects, how we touch other people and how they touch us (if they do touch is a mirror image of our relationship with our own body. When we are tender, gentle and mindful of the messages that our body touches us with -

- *We are in communion with our body.*
- *We are listening to the messages our body is communicating.*
- *We know what is required to move into a place of full recovery - a place where symptoms cannot rear their ugly head.*

Once we are mindful and loving and attentive and appreciative of all the messages our body touches us with, we are solidly on the road to recovery. When we remain detached, distant and uncommunicative with the messages that our body sends to us, we are out of touch and disconnected. In this empty place of disconnection there is little opportunity for true healing to unfold. We are detached from the signals our body so desperately wants us to receive and acknowledge.

Get in touch with your body. Be receptive to its messages. Welcome them. Your body gives to you the information you need to recover. You simply have to be in touch with it.

Come into your full power by getting in touch with your body. Getting in touch with your body is the secret to manifesting your destiny. The world is patiently waiting for you to show your full power.

Make it happen now. Be sensitive to touch. Be aware of the signals. Become intimately compassionate with the moment to moment messages your body sends to you. You are continuously in touch with your body whether you acknowledge it or not. No one succeeds with taking a vacation from your body. Maybe you can take a vacation from work or a spouse. But, you can never take a vacation from your body. Why not become better acquainted? Allow yourself to be touched by its wisdom.

44

Has your work on these exercises been stress free? Has it been helpful in reducing your symptoms? I certainly hope so! This is the primary reason I developed the mindfulness exercises in the first place.

If you struggled with pacing out these mindfulness exercises so as not to induce more stress, there are several Parkinsons Recovery programs that might help expedite your recovery. My Parkinsons Recovery Mindfulness Program sends the mindfulness exercises in an email to you each and every week. The initial exercise is sent to your email address on day one of the week and the deeper implications are sent four days later. The Parkinsons Recovery Mindfulness Program takes one full year to complete as each exercise is introduced one week at a time. For more information visit:

www.stress.parkinsonsrecovery.com

Parkinsons Recovery Memberships involve a variety of support websites that are essential to recovery. A difference mindfulness exercise is posted each week. For more information on Parkinsons Recovery memberships visit:

www.parkinsonsrecovery.org

Of course, the approach that works for many people is to purchase a single volume of the Parkinsons Recovery

Mindfulness program at a time as you have already done! See the introduction for a listing of all nine Parkinsons Recovery Mindfulness volumes.

Thank you for Your Support

On behalf of the thousands of followers of Parkinsons Recovery, I want to thank you for your purchase of this booklet. One hundred percent (100%) of the profits purchases of my books and programs help subsidize the many free services I offer through Parkinsons Recovery -

www.parkinsonsrecovery.com

For information about other products, services and programs visit -

www.parkinsonsrecovery.me